ANTY INFLAMMATORY DIET FOR BEGINNERS

Find Out How to Prep a 21-day Action Plan that Reduces Inflammation, Improve Your Overall Health and Feel Better than Ever, Without Giving Up Taste (Part 1)

BY
Maisie Hamilton

Table of Contents

© Copyright 2020 - All rights reserved.

author is not engaging in the rendering of legal, financial, medical or professional advice. The content within this book has been derived from various sources. Please consult a licensed professional before attempting any techniques outlined in this book.

By reading this document, the reader agrees that under no circumstances is the author responsible for any losses, direct or indirect, which are incurred as a result of the use of information contained within this document, including, but not limited to, — errors, omissions, or inaccuracies.

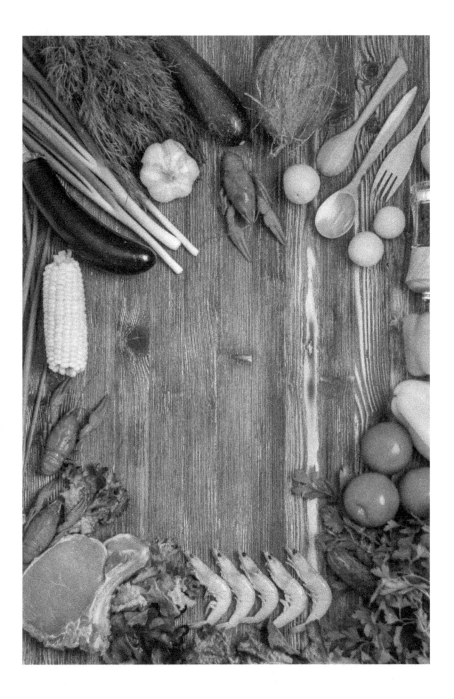

Introduction

To understand why anti-inflammatory diets are so effective at wading off the risk of certain diseases and generally revitalizing your life, you first need to understand what inflammation is, why it is needed, and when it becomes dangerous.

Inflammation is a complex process and it can be of two kids: acute inflammation and chronic. Inflammation is one of the body's natural and most effective defenses against infection of pathogens such as viruses, bacteria, and injury to cells. From infancy, all people become acquainted with the symptoms of inflammation. The word 'symptoms' creates the impression of something scary, which should be avoided but inflammation is a good thing as it is a sign that your body is healing itself.

Acute inflammation occurs frequently and occurs where the body naturally heals itself through the inflammatory process. If you have ever had sprained your ankle or went in for a vaccine, you would have noticed swelling, warmth, and pain around the affected area. Be thankful that this occurred because this is the process of inflammation at work.

But what happens when the body goes haywire and does not know how to control this process? What happens when the body starts attacking itself with a process meant to protect? The answer: damage to the body.

Just like with conditions such as asthma and eczema, the body can become overzealous with its need to protect itself and thus cause more damage than good. This is the case when chronic inflammation occurs. While acute inflammation is an effective protective mechanism that the body has developed to get itself back to working at its optimal conditions as fast as possible in case of injury or infection, chronic inflammation persists over a longer period of time, often not clearing in the correct manner. This causes harm to tissues and cells, and can become so severe that medical intervention is needed, and even then there may not be much that the sufferer can do to reverse the symptoms. The problem is so severe that that chronic inflammation is a disease and has become one of the greatest contributing factors to some of today's most other common chronic diseases. Heart disease, autoimmune dysfunctions, obesity, Alzheimer's disease, and even some forms of cancer are a result of chronic inflammation.

You Can Fight the Debilitating Symptoms of Chronic Inflammation With A Few Simple Changes to Your Diet and Lifestyle

One of the most powerful weapons you can use to fight any of the diseases that are rampant today is knowledge and the same is true with chronic inflammation. This book aims to provide you with the understanding of how chronic inflammation works, what causes it, and what you can do to reduce the effects if it becomes a problem in your life.

Today's society has promoted quick fixes and instant gratification for most problems. However, one cannot slap a bandage on chronic inflammation. Most drugs such as ibuprofen for pain relief only offer a short-term solution. There are even special anti-inflammatory prescription drugs offered to sufferers, but they do not take away the cause of the problem. As a result, the inflammation will persist.

Instead, chronic inflammation needs long-term and strategic solutions, and one of these is making changes to your diet and lifestyle. The reason that diet is such an important contributing factor to decreasing the problem of chronic inflammation is because many of the foods that we eat and drink everyday introduce toxins into our bodies. The body then tries to attack and eliminate these toxins by increasing the instances of inflammation. In addition to causing the flare-up of inflammation, these toxins contribute toward a number of other health problems, hence the epidemic that is widespread with an increasing number of obesity and heart disease cases, and a myriad of other health issues worldwide.

Processed food is one of the most dangerous to consume yet most people do so daily. Everyday we introduce artificial ingredients, bad carbohydrates, large amounts of sugar, and many more harmful ingredients to the body. It is no wonder that inflammation and the other associated diseases are on the rise. The convenience of these foods is clearly overshadowed by the fact that they are addictive and use the body as dumping ground for toxins.

Control Inflammation to Improve Your Overall Health

Your body is a temple. You only get one body. Therefore, you should do everything in your power to ensure that you care for it in the best way possible. General health and wellness are directly related to eating habits.

The age old saying of "You are what you eat," is as true today as it was a century ago. By taking control of what you eat, when you eat it, and how you eat it, you can control the way you look, feel, and think.

If you consume processed foods and foods high in sugar but skimp on your veggies and fruits, it will be reflected in your waistline, probably in the acne on your cheeks and even in the luster of your hair. But the problems are not limited to your physical appearance. In fact, the external signs of a poor diet are normally just a glimpse of what is going on within.

By eating clean, wholesome, and fresh foods, you can control how your body deposits fat, how it detoxes itself and the amount of detoxification it goes through, it has to do and the good nutrients it has available. The internal conditions of your body will thrive and it will reflect in the outer appearance of your body. Your will like become slimmer, have healthier skin and fuller hair. You will also improve your mental and emotional states, promoting a happier, more fulfilled you.

Most often, controlling chronic inflammation is as easy as controlling your diet. Participating in an anti inflammatory diet detoxifies the body and helps facilitate the healing process in a healthy way. The widespread benefits of practicing an anti inflammatory diet on the inflammation process and general health and wellness are not just hearsay. Medical research and studies have repeatedly shown that an anti inflammatory diet protects the body against many acute and chronic diseases including chronic inflammation. The diet does this by enhancing the metabolic processes of the body as well as stabilizing blood sugar and cholesterol levels, all processes that promote an overall healthy individual.

There are no disadvantages to practicing an anti inflammatory diet even if you do not suffer from chronic inflammation. While this book is meant to provide you with the knowledge that you need to fight chronic inflammation in a practical, actionable way, it is also meant to show you that this diet, along with other lifestyle such as a proper exercise regiment, can allow you to achieve your health goals in a painless, progresive way.

The pages to come are information-packed and founded on sound studies and sources. You will learn more on the differences between acute and chronic inflammation, how to prepare your body for an anti inflammatory diet, the foods you should eat and those you should avoid to decrease the likelihood of chronic inflammation, and those that are most effective in promoting the production of pro-inflammatory substances within the body. In addition, you will be given over 100 recipes for breakfast, lunch, dinner, and everything in between to make this a tasty journey for you as well. The included information on grocery shopping and the food pyramid depicting recommended serving sizes and nutritional values will also help you experiment and create your own recipes that do not undo the hard work you have put into reaping the rewards of this diet.

This is a guidebook and cookbook combined into one powerful source of all things inflammation! And best yet, the information has been assimilated for an easy-to-read, seamless flow using terminology that that anyone can understand.

Turn to the next page to better understand inflammation and how it affects your daily life, to change your outlook on your diet for overall wellness and to improve your diet so that your can live happier, healthier, and more holistically.

Chapter 1:
What Is Inflammation?

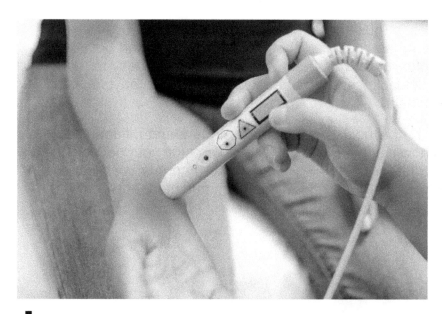

I n the introductory chapter, we supplied the basic definition what inflammation is. however, the process is more in-depth and far more complicated than the surface signs that we see. Inflammation one of the body's first lines of defense in response to injury, trauma or infection. It is a signal that the immune system needs to repair and heal damaged tissue as well as put up a line of defense against foreign entities such as bacteria and viruses. This process is facilitated by the presence of white blood cells and other substances that protect the body come foreign or outside invaders. In essence, the body unleashes a mini army to clear out any malevolent invaders. This army release is facilitated by chemical signals that tell the white blood cells aka the soldiers in this army, where to stand and when to start fighting.

In addition to all these complex advantages, inflammation also limits the area where tissue is damaged and stops the spread of foreign microbes as to minimize the damage caused. Inflammation also clears away any debris that is created from the process so that the tissue can heal in a clean and safe environment.

Without this physiological line of defense, wounds would not heal and instead they would fester. Without this defense, infections would overrun the body and become deadly. Without inflammation, the human population will dwindle down to nothing.

What Happens When Inflammation Goes on for Too Long?

There are two types of inflammation. The first is called acute inflammation it is a short-term response to the site of a problem such as a cut on the knee, burn, broken bone or scraped flesh. symptoms include:

- Pain
- Redness
- Swelling
- Heat at the site of the existing problem
- Loss of function at the site

When acute inflammation occurs, the body responds by dilating blood vessels to increase blood flow to the site of the problem. At the site of injury or infection, tissue in need of aid releases a chemical called cytokines which signal the need for white blood cells to the injured or infected area to promote healing. Nutrients are also delivered to the site to aid in the healing process.

Substances called prostaglandins are also released at the site. They promote blood clotting to heal damaged tissue and cause pain and fever, both of which are signs that the healing process has been activated.

As the body heals, the symptoms of inflammation gradually subside and cease altogether. Pain, redness, swelling, and the other common symptoms of inflammation stop. After cells have regenerated themselves and tissue has healed itself, the site of inflammation is restored to a normal appearance. Blood flow resumes to normal and white blood cells return to their normal levels and functions within the body.

It is not only physical injury that activates acute inflammation. Radiation, chemical irritants, and toxins also cause an instant flare-up of inflammation depending on the level of exposure and hazardousness. Infection of bacteria, viruses, and other foreign pathogens also cause inflammation although there may be a delay in the show of symptoms as the attack on the body occurs internally rather than from the outside. A common example of this is a sore throat. To make the process of acute inflammation clearer in your mind, let's break it down into the individual steps:

1. A harmful stimulus such as a cut or pathogens are detected by the body.
2. Cells belonging to the immune system at the site of the infected tissue become active. Their receptors detected the damage or invasion. They then release chemicals that dilate blood vessels nearby to increase blood flow to the site.
3. This increased blood flow brings white blood cells to the site. Glucose, which is a sugar, and oxygen are

also delivered to the site. They nourish the cells there, increasing their ability to repair and heal the damaged tissue. As a result of the blood vessel dilation, plasma proteins and antibodies are also delivered to the site.

4. Swelling, heat, pain, and redness occur at the site because of the above conditions and reactions. Even more white blood cells are delivered, especially if a pathogenic infection is the cause of this process activation. These cells not only destroy the pathogens, they also help repair any wounds. The presence of white blood cells also wards off any further attacks from pathogens.

5. Once the pathogens have been isolated, cleanup commences. Dead cells, both internal and invasive, and other debris created in the healing process are removed from the site. New cells replace the old ones and excess white blood cells leave the area. Once all of this is done, everything at the site returns to normal.

This a smooth process but sometimes there is a breakdown in this process, which is what occurs with the other type of inflammation.

Chronic Inflammation and Why it is Harmful

Remember the old saying that "Too much of a good thing is bad?" This saying applies in this case as well. Inflammation can go on for too long or can occur in places where it is not needed. This is what occurs in the second form of inflammation, which is called chronic inflammation. This type of inflammation is also called persistent, low-grade inflammation because it occurs over a prolonged of time unlike acute inflammation which usually persists for a few days or less. Chronic inflammation can persist for years and causes cellular destruction, scar tissue, fibrosis, and abscess formation to occur. This condition is a disease and needs to be treated at the earliest to avoid the negative consequences. Referring to the smooth process outlined above in the case of acute inflammation, chronic inflammation often breakdowns at the termination phase of the process. In fact, the process does not stop and one reason for this is that white blood cells and other chemicals released by the immune system periodically check cells for normailities. If all is normal, then they terminate the inflammation process. With chronic inflammation, the immune system cells mistake normal body cells for harmful cells and continue attacking at the site. It destroys the cells, thus harming the body rather than curing it. Chronic inflammation is harmful on its own but the dangers only increase as it has been linked to several diseases. Some of these common diseases are cardiovascular diseases such as stroke or heart disease and autoimmune disorders like lupus, rheumatoid arthritis, gouty arthritis, and psoriatic arthritis. Cancer is another disease that has been linked to this condition as it causes damage of DNA, thus giving rise to abnormalities. The cancers that may be a result of inflammation include colon cancer, breast cancer, and colorectal cancer.

Chronic inflammation is often characterized by symptoms such as:

- Joint pain
- Joint stiffness
- Loss of brain function
- Swollen joints that can be warm to the touch

While these listed above are the most common symptoms of chronic inflammation, some people may experience flu-like symptoms as well. These include:

- Headaches
- Chills

- Fever
- Muscle stiffness
- Loss of appetite
- Fatigue

Other unusual symptoms include chronic diarrhea and numbness to one side of the face.

What Causes Chronic Inflammation?

Inflammation can be caused by any number of physical, biological, chemical, psychological, and environmental factors. As a result of these factors, there are people who are at greater risk of developing chronic inflammation. By being informed about these, you can first evaluate yourself for these risk factors then take the appropriate steps to prevent chronic inflammation.

Those Most At Risk For Chronic Inflammation

They are:

- People who have suffered from blunt or penetrating physical injuries like frostbite and burns.
- People who are overweight or obese. This is due to the fact that the body naturally attacks fat deposits as they are mistaken for foreign entities. This causes the fat cells to break, resulting in leakages activate the inflammation process.
- People with a history of heart disease or heart disease in the family.
- People with type 2 diabetes. This is a two-fold process as people with this type of diabetes normally develop inflammation while people with chronic inflammation typically develop type 2 diabetes.
- People who frequent toxic environments.

- People who suffer from chronic fatigue.
- People who suffer from high levels of stress or mental disorders like depression.
- Older people. This is because human beings tend to release more chemicals that promote inflammation and less of anti-inflammatory chemicals as they get older.

How is Chronic Inflammation Diagnosed?

Chronic inflammation is diagnosed by testing the blood for certain indicators. Such indicators include:

- The existence of the protein molecule called cytokine. This molecule is secreted to regulate the immune system. There are two types of cytokines and they are called tumor necrosis factor alpha (TNFa) and interleukin-6 (IL-6). IL-6 is the one to look out for as it is a proinflammatory chemical and triggers the initial phases of acute inflammation.
- High levels of CRP (C-reactive protein). CRP is produced in the liver in response to inflammation.
- Analysis through serum protein electrophoresis (SPE). This is a measure of certain proteins in blood cells. Too much and too little of these particular proteins can signal inflammation in addition to other conditions.
- Analysis of the Erythrocyte Sedimentation Rate (ESR). This blood test measures the rate at which red blood cells sink in a tube of blood. If they sink quickly, this can be an indicator of inflammation. This taste is called a sedimentation rate test and is usually done in conjunction with other tests.
- The thickness of blood. Inflammation can cause the blood to thicken.

There are other diagnostic tests that can be done and these include:

- Colonoscopy
- Sigmoidoscopy
- Upper endoscopy

These are tests on the digestive tract.

X-rays and MRIs can also be performed to check certain parts of the body upon request by doctors.

Chapter 2:
Anti-Inflammatory Diets and How They
Can Improve Your Overall Health

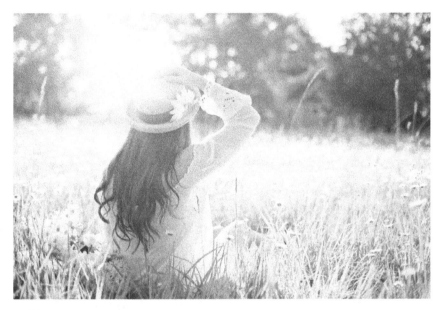

D iets have become all the rage these days with fancy names and outrageous meal plans and unusual recipes. The anti inflammatory diet is not a fancy term nor does it require any off the wall recipes to work. In fact, I would go so far as to say that it is not even a particular diet, but a variety of other diets combined to develop a comprehensive eating plan that optimizes the way your body works.

Types of Eating Regimens to Reduce Chronic Inflammation

Mediterranean Diet

This eating regimen is inspired by the eating habits of people who live in the Mediterrean region. This eating regimen consists of a high consumption of olive oil, fruits, vegetables, legumes, and unrefined grains in addition to seafood and dairy products like cheese and yogurt. Red meats are resisted in the preparation of Mediterranean meals. There is also a great emphasis on the consumption of wine!

This eating regimen is a great addition to the anti inflammatory diet because it reduces inflammatory indicators such as IL-6 and CRP because of is beneficial injection of dietary fibers and monounsaturated fats into the diet while keeping saturated fats low.

The other health benefits of this eating regimen include lowering the rates of neurodegeneration, certain chronic diseases, cardiovascular diseases, and reducing the risk of cancer. These benefits are largely due to the use of olive oil because of its anti inflammatory benefits due to the presence of a fatty acid called oleic acid. Olive oil also contains antioxidants, which are substances that removes potentially damaging oxidizing agents from the body, helps prevent cardiovascular disease and is not associated with weight gain despite being an oil.

Vegetarian and Vegan Diets

These two eating regimens consist of principally plant-based foods which are rich in vitamin K. Dark, green, and leafy vegetables like spinach, kale, and broccoli are largely used in these two types of eating plans. They have long been known to fight the symptoms of chronic inflammation.

Fruits are also a big part of these two eating plans. Colorful fruits such as blackberries and raspberries are particularly helpful in fighting inflammation as the pigment that produces their vibrant colors contains a vital substance for fighting the symptoms.

In addition, these regimens promote the use of vegan protein sources and fish instead of red meat. Combined, all of these components aid in increasing the levels of plasma amino acid, which is an indicator of lowered risk of inflammation and by extension, heart disease.

Low Carb Eating Diet

The title is largely self-explanatory and not only does it help reduce the instances of chronic inflammation, but it also helps to reduce other health issues such as high blood pressure, diabetes, cardiovascular diseases, and many digestive issues. The principal of this eating regiment entails replacing easily digestible low-carb foods such as bread, rice, sugar, and pasta with foods that are rich in fats yet moderate in proteins. These replacements usually come in the form of seafood, nuts, and seeds, dairy, dark green leafy vegetables or fruits.

There are several low carb diets out there but some of the most effective at helping fight inflammation are the ketogenic diet, the Atkins diet, and the paleo diet all of which are based on a low carb intake.

Eating for Better Health and Anti Inflammation

Foods that Increase the Risk of Chronic Inflammation and that Should be Avoided

As a general rule of thumb, anything that is highly processed, overly sweet, greasy, and packaged can increase your risk of developing chronic inflammation. You may be tempted to reach for them when you go to the supermarket, but muster up that resistance to do so. In fact, they should be completely crossed off from your shopping list and meal plans.

To make it even easier, here is a comprehensive list of the foods that should be avoided in order to reduce the risk of developing chronic inflammation.

Red meats that have been processed and contain high fats

Example of these includes hot dogs and sausages. They contain high amounts of saturated fats, something which has been shown to directly cause inflammation.

Processed whole milk, cheese, and butter

These have a high saturated fat content. Only low-fat dairy products should be consumed.

Fried foods

While the body does need a moderate amount of fatty acids, consuming foods that have been fried in vegetable oil such as corn oil increases the amount of omega-6 fatty acids in the body. The increase in omega-6 fatty acids may disturb the amount of Omega-3 fatty acids and this imbalance gives rise to inflammatory problems.

Foods that contain trans fats

Trans fats also known as trans fatty acids are derived from solid fats which have been converted from liquid vegetable oil in a process called hydrogenation. Trans fats increase the levels of low-density lipoproteins (LDL) which is a bad cholesterol and which causes the flare-up of inflammation. Even products on your grocery shelf that carry a partially hydrogenated fat or oil in the ingredient list should be avoided even if it is just minute traces of trans fat.

Refined carbohydrates

Refined carbohydrates differ from unrefined carbohydrates in that they are process to remove a lot of the natural nutrition resulting in a loss of essential vitamins and minerals. Common refined carbohydrates include white bread and white pasta. Due to their high sugar and carbohydrate components, they cause the body to release cytokines which is an inflammatory agent. Not only do they increase the risk of chronic inflammation but they cause weight gain, high cholesterol levels, and high blood sugar conditions which are bad for overall health and wellness.

Sweetened foods and beverages

Foods that contain a high amount of sugars, such as soda, fruit juices, and sugary snacks should be avoided. Even honey and agave cause flare-ups in inflammation.

Glutinous grains

Gluten is the substance that is generated when water is mixed with water soluble proteins found in wheat and green flowers. gluten has been shown to aggravate inflammation therefore grains such as wheat, rye and barley should be avoided.

Nightshades

Nightshades are mostly comprised of plants, shrubs, and herbs that are poisonous, but some edible fruits such as potatoes and eggplant, which are safe to eat stimulate chronic inflammation.

Foods that are Good to Eat

Fruits and Vegetables

By consuming these, you stock up on the essential vitamins, minerals, and antioxidants the body needs to support the immune system and thus reduce chronic inflammation. Deeply colored fruit varieties like raspberries, grapes, oranges, blackberries, and fruits that are high in good fats like olives and avocados are the best choice. Many berries contain the antioxidant called anthocyanin, which offers anti inflammatory, antiviral and anti cancer benefits.

As for veggies, reach for the dark, green leafy types first. These include collard greens, kale, spinach, and broccoli to name a few. Broccoli in particular is rich in sulforaphane, an antioxidant that helps reduce cytokine levels to fight inflammation.

To gain the best nutrition out of these, adults should consume up to two cups of fresh fruit three times daily and three cups of organic vegetables four times daily.

Unrefined Whole Grains

Get your essential vitamins and iron from consuming these. Not only are you benefitting from the nutritional value, but there are several other benefits such as reducing cholesterol levels through the stabilization of blood sugar levels, aiding in weight loss management by suppressing the hormones that trigger hunger signals, and it also helps circulate oxygen-rich red blood cells throughout the entire body. Consuming unrefined whole grains such as whole grain or multigrain bread that has been sweetened with fruit sweeteners such as raisins, brown rice, and unrefined cereal grains like quinoa and bulgur also help lower your risk of developing cardiovascular disease. Adults should consume unrefined whole grains four times a day.

Nuts and Seeds

Nuts like almonds, cashew nuts, peanuts, Brazil nuts, walnuts, and pistachios, and seeds like chia seeds, pumpkin seeds, and ground flaxseed contain healthy monounsaturated fats, fiber, and protein to help you lose weight and control inflammation as long as they are consumed in moderation. No more than a handful or 1.5 ounces should be consumed daily by adults. Other notable nuts include hazelnuts and pine nuts and nutritious seeds include hemp and sesame seeds.

Fatty Fish

These include tuna, sardines, herring, cod, salmon, anchovies, and mackerel. They contain omega-3 fatty acids that lower IL-6 and CRP quantities to reduce the incidence of inflammation. Fatty fish should be consumed between twice and six times a week in quantities of around 4 ounces.

Healthy Herbs and Spices

Use less salt and add flavor to your food the natural and safe way. You can stock up your spice cabinets with the following herbs and spices to not only make your food taste great but to prevent chronic inflammation:

- Ginger, which can be used in both sweet and savory dishes, contains the antioxidant gingerol, which packs quite the punch to reduce many gastrointestinal disorders and to treat the pain of rheumatoid arthritis.
- Turmeric contains a chemical called curcumin. This helps fight other conditions related to chronic inflammation such as Alzheimer's disease and arthritis. Turmeric is most effective when combined with black pepper because it is absorbed by the body better. This is what gives curry powder its vibrant color.

- Garlic contains an anti inflammatory compound that inhibits proinflammatory compounds such as cytokines. It also helps relieve pain and fights against cartilage damage caused by arthritis.
- Cinnamon has antioxidant properties. In addition to its aid in anti inflammation, it helps the body repair damage done to cells by free radicals.
- Sweet and spicy peppers help reduce inflammation and relieve pain because they contain capsaicin compounds. Bell peppers and chilli peppers are packed with antioxidants and vitamin C, both of which promote anti inflammation.

Beans and Legumes

This food group includes red kidney beans, garbanzos, chickpeas, lentils, and black beans. They are rich in antioxidants, good fats, fiber, iron, zinc, potassium, folate, and magnesium, all of which are anti inflammatory substances. It is great to consume one cup of beans and legumes two times a day.

Soy

Soy-based foods are a great source of fiber, which help keep your digestive system in good working order. These foods should be consumed once or twice daily and include items such as tofu, soybeans, soy flour, soymilk, soy nuts, and tempeh.

Natural Teas

It is a great idea to consume natural teas such as green, black, white, and ginger about three times a day. These help protect the body from several diseases, many of which are associated with chronic inflammation. They have this power because they are steeped in polyphenols. Teas are also a great source of antioxidants, which helps fight chronic inflammation. Green tea contains a substance called EGCCG (epigallocatechin-3-gallate), which reduces cytokine levels.

Red Wine

This contains a compound called resveratrol, which is an anti inflammatory substance. It also contains antioxidants to protect the body from certain cancers and cardiovascular disease. One of the most widely talked about benefits of red wine are its anti aging properties. When consumed in moderation that is. The recommended daily serving is five ounces or less for women and 10 ounces or less for men.

Certain Sweets

If you have a sweet tooth, do not fear. Not all sweets are banned from the anti inflammatory diet. Select sweets such as plain dark chocolate and plant-based syrups like maple syrup and fruit sugars are allowed. Dark chocolate in packed with antioxidants. Ensure that if you indulge in this sweet that it has at least 70% cocoa to enjoy the most anti inflammatory benefits.

Anti Inflammatory Supplements

Common supplements used to fight chronic inflammation include garlic, fish oils, and onions. However, you can boost the benefits of these by also taking berberine, spirulina, ALA (alpha lipoic acid), and curcumin.

Berberine is a tonic supplement. Extracted from goldenseal or barberry plants, it helps treat gastrointestinal problems such as IBS (irritable bowel syndrome) and UC (ulcerative colitis) which is inflammation of the colon, is an antibacterial agent and also helps reduce fever. This supplement also helps lower blood sugar levels.

Spirulina is a probiotic and helps promote the growth and balance of good bacteria in the gut. It is obtained from blue-green algae called cyanobacteria. This supplement is rich in vitamins A and B12 as well as some minerals and proteins. These help reduce chronic inflammation and the resulting negative effects.

ALA helps eliminate heavy metals such as mercury, lead, and copper, which can be harmful, from the bloodstream. It is an antioxidant and healthy fatty acid.

Curcumin helps reduce fever and is a natural pain reliever.

A Helpful Shopping List

It is always a good idea to keep your cabinets and refrigerator stocked with the good stuff that will help you fight inflammation rather than promote it. Below you can find anti inflammatory products that you can find at most grocery stores. These make a good compliment to the items already listed above.

Fruits

Grapefruits, bananas, cucumbers, apples, lemons, limes, mangoes, pomegranates, peaches, strawberries, cherries, blueberries, tomatoes, and watermelon.

Vegetables

Bok choy, cauliflower, Brussels sprouts, pumpkin, romaine lettuce, mushrooms, and yellow onions.

Unrefined Whole Grains

Rolled oatmeal, barley, and brown rice

Fatty Fish

Trout, albacore tuna.

Herbs and Spices

All-spice, basil, bay leaf, black pepper, caraway seeds, cardamom, cayenne, cloves, coriander, cumin, dill, fennel, lemongrass, mint, nutmeg, oregano, paprika, rosemary, sage, tarragon, and thyme.

Natural Teas

Dandelion, cherry, ginger, masala chai, oolong, pineapple, rooibos, rosehips, and turmeric,

Sweets and Sweeteners

Sweetener with low glycemic indexes like stevia and allulose, erythritol

Others

Baking powder, peanut butter

Chapter 3:
Preparing to Practice the Anti Inflammatory Diet

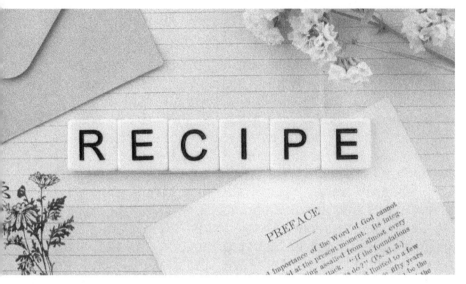

M ost people fail at dieting not because it is hard to do but because they did not mentally prepare or set goals when they began the regimen. By taking the time to set your goals and plan the way forward, you pave the way to keep focused and motivated when the going gets tough, which it eventually will. You create a sense of purpose and have a vision of what you would like to achieve. Is it simply enough to live a healthy lifestyle and prevent common illness and disease? Perhaps you would like to lose weight in combination with decreasing inflammation triggers in your diet? Maybe it is because you want to decrease your chances of developing heart disease?

No matter what you would like to achieve, setting a goal that is smart, measurable, realistic, and irrelevant sets you up for success. Sticking to a diet of any kind involves developing good habits to replace your bad habits. For example, instead of reaching for French fries as a snack, fill up on fruits and vegetables. The longer you practice this, the more likely you are to do it like it's second nature in the future. After a while, you will not even think about the benefits or need to keep yourself motivated to reach for the healthier alternative. It will simply become muscle memory.

Hold yourself accountable and monitor your progress. Journaling is a great way to do this as it shows you how far you have come. Every small step contributes toward your greater success. Sometimes the small steps are unclear in your mind at first, however, when you create a system where you can see their contribution and track them, you can realize their relevance. Lose 20 lb in one week! Many of us have heard many an advertisement promoting achievements that seemed impossible if done in a healthy way. While it is certainly possible to lose 20 lb in one week, it is most often involves starving the body and creating unhealthy conditions internally. Undertaking such an endeavor creates more harm than good. Do not get caught up in the hype. Set goals that are realistic and do not put unnecessary or harmful demands on your body. This will help keep you motivated and avoid false starts.

Also plan for setbacks. No matter what area of your life that you set goals for, there will be roadblocks and hurdles to face. Do not feel dejected or let this hinder your progress in any way. Consider the possible setbacks and have a plan to get you back on track as quickly as possible should they occur. In addition to setting your goals, allow time to reassess and adjust your goals if it is needed. I am saying this not to overwhelm you, but to impress upon you the importance of developing the right mindset to not only eat healthier, but to completely overhaul your life for a physical, mental, and emotional transformation. It is not enough to change your diet, even as important as that aspect is. To get the most out of anti inflammation diet, you need to change your lifestyle.

It might seem hard at first, especially if you suffer from sugar addiction which we will cover a little later on in this chapter, but I guarantee you that the benefits will be worth it in the end.

Sugar and Its Effects on Inflammation

Sugar is a known trigger for chronic information as it promotes the secretion of inflammatory indicators such as CRP and the production of LDL cholesterol, which is known as the bad cholesterol.

In addition to its negative contribution to chronic inflammation, sugar can lead to weight gain, digestive issues, heart disease, type 2 diabetes, liver disease and even some types of cancers.

With so many negative effects, it is obvious that sugar intake needs to be limited and quite possibly eliminated from the diet to ensure good health and longevity. However, removing sugar from their diet can be very difficult for most of the global population.

How to Deal with Sugar Withdrawal

Sugar is eight times as addictive as cocaine. Is it any wonder that most people cannot just stop consuming it even though they know how damaging it is to their health when consumed in unhealthy amounts? You may not even realize that you have a sugar dependency because you do not consume a lot of foods that are considered high in sugar. However, there are many foods that contain hidden sugars. Examples of this include granola bars, yogurt, crackers, pasta sauce, salad dressings, breakfast cereals, and instant oatmeal.

Excessive sugar intake has been linked to obesity, heart disease, cancer, type 2 diabetes, poor dental health, and more. The reason sugar is so addictive is that it creates a cycle of chronic craving because it gives a rush of energy when consumed. That rush is quickly followed by a sudden drop in energy. Your body craves that high again and therefore, craves sugar. This creates an endless cycle if you do not put a stop to it.

Let's take a closer look at how this addictive cycle works:

1. You consume a sugary food.
2. Insulin levels become elevated and your liver converts sugar into fat.
3. When this sugar enters your bloodstream, your blood pressure rises.
4. The levels of dopamine, a feel-good hormone, increases and makes you feel happy, working similarly to how heroin does.
5. Due to the high levels of insulin, sugar levels fall rapidly, hence, creating a feeling of fatigue. This sends signals to your brain making it crave for more sugar.
6. Therefore, you consume more sugary foods.

Excessive sugar intake is not only a trigger for inflammation, it also:

- Causes bad breath and dental cavities as it promotes the development of bacteria in the mouth.

- Causes skin to age faster since it attaches itself to collagen proteins to create AGEs also known as advanced glycation end products, which causes skin to lose its elasticity hereby creating wrinkles
- Increases the risk of developing type 2 diabetes and heart disease as it causes the pancreas to work overtime to pump out insulin which breaks down the organ.
- Increases the risk of kidney damage as the kidneys need to filter blood sugar levels.
- Make blood vessels to grow faster than normal and get tense, which creates a narrow space for blood to travel. This increases the stress on the heart and therefore elevates the risk of developing heart disease.

Sugar is a simple carbohydrate molecule, however, its effects on our bodies are rather significant. As sugar is a carbohydrate, in addition to the unhealthy dependency it creates, it is a substance that is not allowed in the anti inflammatory diet. If you are like most of the world population, you too might suffer from a sugar dependency and as such you should expect to feel the symptoms that come with the withdrawal from it. Remember that this is more addicting that cocaine.

Sugar withdrawal symptoms include:

- Headaches
- Decreased energy
- Lowered mental acuteness
- Gastrointestinal distress

The important thing to remember is that this is a temporary phase. In a few days, you will get relief as long as you stick with the diet.

Most people think that we need sugar in our diets but fundamentally we do not. Sugar is an energy source. We can replace it with better alternatives that treat our bodies better. Proteins and fats are more powerful sources of energy. While they may not be as quick to breakdown and produce that rush of energy, their effect is more sustainable and healthier for the gut. Protein and fat can be obtained from fatty fish, fruits, vegetables, seeds, and nuts.

The anti inflammatory diet helps detox sugar from your lifestyle. You do this by removing substances from your cabinets and repairing your eating habits. While it may at first be difficult to keep away from the sugary temptation, think of the benefits in addition to the obvious of fight against chronic inflammation. They include:

- Weight loss
- Reduced bloating
- More regulated moods
- Better dental health
- Sustained energy through the day
- Clearer skin.

Helpful Lifestyle Tips on Managing Chronic Inflammation

Remember that to fight chronic inflammation, it is not enough to just change your diet. You also need to make changes in your life that will not only fight inflammation, but will also help you fight other diseases, enjoy general good health and wellness, and make you a happier, more fulfilled individual. Some solutions for living a healthy lifestyle that fights chronic inflammation are included below:

Count Calories For Better Health

Counting calories has traditionally been a way to help people lose weight. By extension, it is also beneficial in preventing the trigger of chronic inflammation. While this is a widely used term, most people only have a vague notion of what it is. Let's take a look at what a calorie actually is before we move further.

A calorie is a measure of energy, specifically the amount of energy in foods. We use it for biological functions in our bodies such as breathing, thinking, walking, and talking. Calories are not bad things as they have been portrayed to be. The issue arises when there is an excessive intake of calories than our personalized recommended intake. The body stores excess calories in the form of fat, leading to weight gain over time. The body views fat deposits as an intrusion, leading to the immune system attacking itself which causes chronic inflammation.

By counting calories, you become more aware of what you are putting into your body and thus increases your chances of managing your weight in an effective and sustainable way. The number of calories you should consume daily depends on factors such as activity level, gender, metabolic health, age, and weight. However, on average, a woman needs 2000 calories a day while a man needs 2500 calories per day.

Most times, the only thing you need to do to control your calorie intake is to lower your portion sizes. However, there are certain foods that provide the body with a lot more calories compared to others.

For the best results when counting calories are a few tips:

- Measure your calorie intake with a mobile app or online, which will help you measure your calorie intake for the food you consume.

- Get rid of the junk food in your cupboards as most of them have high calorie counts. Replace them with healthy alternatives such as fruits, nuts, seeds, and vegetables.
- Read the labels on the food you purchase as most of them contain useful nutritional information including the calorie count per serving.
- Consume enough calories to fuel your workout or exercise regiment as dieting and exercise go hand-in-hand.
- Do not try to undercut your calorie intake as consuming too few calories will leave you feeling fatigued throughout the day.

To help you get the most out of the calories that you consume from the recipes to come in the following chapters, we have included the calorie count.

Exercising and its Anti Inflammatory Benefits

Exercising is an effective way of fighting inflammation in addition to its many benefits such as reducing the risk of developing cardiovascular disease, type 2 diabetes, and some forms of cancer. Exercise also helps lower blood pressure, improve metabolism, and control weight loss.

Several studies have shown that just 20 minutes of exercise per day helps reduce the production of pro inflammation indicators such as cytokines and CRP. Exercise also makes your body muscle release protein called IL-6 (Interleukin 6), which has many anti-inflammatory effects such as:

- Decreasing the levels of a protein called TNF alpha, which is a pro inflammation substance.
- Inhibiting the signaling effects of a protein called interleukin 1 beta. This protein triggers inflammation.

How long you exercise is directly proportional to how much you will benefit from the anti-inflammatory properties of IL -6. The longer you exercise, the more of this substance is released. This protein's levels peak at the time that you finish your workout and rapidly decreases back to its pre-existing levels. However, the effects are long-lasting in preventing the trigger of inflammation.

How Stress Contributes Toward Chronic Inflammation and How you can Manage it

We live in a fast-paced world and avoiding stress is next to impossible. Most people feel tired, distracted, irritated, and plagued with the feeling that they are not doing enough everyday. Most people think that this is simply part of daily living and do not realize the deep impact that stress has on the development of several diseases such as cardiovascular disease, type 2 diabetes and autoimmune disorders.

Extensive stress also triggers chronic inflammation.

Stress triggers a fight or flight response, which is a short-term survival response that evolution has programmed within us to keep us safe. This response triggers the release of several hormones, such as adrenaline and cortisol. Cortisol has been dubbed the stress hormone and it promotes inflammation. Therefore by remaining in a near-constant state of stress, you are essentially triggering chronic inflammation within your body.

A few ways to help manage your stress levels are by:

- Practicing meditation.
- Not multitasking. Instead, focus on one thing at a time.
- Taking a break from what you are doing if you feel overwhelmed, taking a full body analysis and identifying what is happening within it and actively bringing yourself back to a calmer, more peaceful state of mind.
- Exercising regularly.
- Getting enough sleep.
- Cultivating a healthier emotional state by practicing gratitude, compassion, and joy.
- Spending more time outdoors.
- Eating nutritious foods.

Managing your stress levels starts within yourself. Take the time to care for your mental and emotional health. Simple changes that you can make in your work and home life can drastically reduce your stress levels and therefore, your risk for several diseases including chronic inflammation.

Why Getting Enough Sleep is Important

Sleep is vital for the proper function of the body physically, emotionally, and mentally. Its many benefits include:

- Increased performance
- Elevated mood
- Improved memory

You are not at your best when your sleep has been disrupted or when you are suffering from a lack of proper sleep. Suffering from chronic inflammation likely results in disturbances in sleep pattern and receiving adequate sleep. Chronic inflammation gives rise to sleeping disorders like sleep apnea, insomnia, and restless leg syndrome.

Inflammation disrupts sleep in the following ways:

- It causes pain, which interferes with sleep.
- It causes stress when it is time to sleep. Chronic inflammation can cause an increase in the levels of cortisol which is a stress hormone, thereby increasing the chances that you will not be able to fall asleep at certain times of the night.
- It affects the sleep center of your brain. This part of your brain is called the hypothalamus. It is responsible for your sleep patterns. Chronic inflammation disrupts the signals in that part of the brain hereby disrupting your ability to fall asleep and stay asleep.
- It causes movement during sleep, which in itself, disrupts sleep. When in pain and discomfort due to chronic inflammation, the sufferer is more likely to move around during sleep time. This constant movement causes the sufferer to wake frequently hereby disrupting his or her sleep patterns.
- It affects the sufferer's ability to achieve rapid eye movement (REM) sleep, which is the part of the sleep cycle where you are in deep sleep, dreaming, and having the utmost rest. During REM sleep, endorphins, pain relief hormones, growth hormones, and healing hormones are released. Therefore, not

being able to achieve REM sleep not only makes you feel less rested, but it also deprives you of these essential hormones.

The flip side of the coin is that bad sleep habits can also contribute toward inflammation. Sleep and inflammation are regulated by the same biological rhythm. We fall asleep and wake to a rhythm called the circadian rhythm. This is driven by the secretion and inhibitions of certain hormones within the 24-hour period. This same circadian rhythm regulates the immune system and thus the inflammation function. Once this rhythm is disrupted, so is the normal function of inflammation. Getting too little sleep and too much sleep trigger inflammation

To maintain a healthy circadian rhythm and thus healthy inflammation, develop and maintain a consistent sleep routine. Go to bed and wake up at the same time everyday while ensuring that you get the right number of hours of rest.

Most adults need between seven and nine hours of sleep every night. A deviation from that amount, for even one day, can trigger inflammation. Just imagine what this does to your body and immune system over a prolonged period of time. This happens because inadequate amounts of sleep cause the rise in pro inflammatory hormones. It is good to note that this effect is more prominent in women than in men.

Now that we have increased your knowledge and awareness of chronic inflammation, its causes and effects, and how we can prevent it, let's move onto those recipes that are not only great for our taste buds and good for our stomach, but also anti inflammatory. We have also included a few helpful notes on the recipes so that you can be assured that you are getting the most anti inflammatory benefits from each recipe.

Chapter 4:
Week 1 Recipes

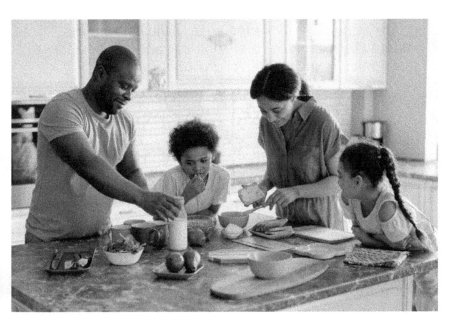

Breakfast

Fluffy Banana Pancakes

Bananas are a great way to restore energy and relieve aches and pains. They contain antioxidants and a special compound called rutin that helps fight inflammation.

Nutritional Information

Calcium	246mg
Dietary Fiber	13g
Iron	6g
Potassium	1326mg
Sodium	166mg
Protein	6.5g
Sugars	54g
Total Carbohydrates	85.2g
Total Fat	23.7g
Calories per serving	187

Time: 20 minutes

Serving Size: 1

Ingredients:

- 1 small firm banana

- ¼ cup of applesauce (pureed cooked apple)
- 1 tablespoon of soy flour
- ⅛ teaspoon of baking powder
- ¼ teaspoon of ground cinnamon
- ⅛ teaspoon of ground nutmeg
- 1 ½ tablespoon of olive oil
- A pinch of salt
- 5 blueberries for topping

Directions:

1. Peel and mash the banana in a bowl.
2. Add the applesauce, baking powder, flour, cinnamon, salt, and nutmeg. Mix well to form a smooth batter.
3. Heat the oil in a large frying pan over medium heat. Add three tablespoons of batter into the frying pan to make 1 pancake. Add as many pancakes as the pan allows.
4. Cook this until small bubbles form on the top of the pancake then flip to cook the other side.
5. The pancakes should be golden brown on each side. Move the pancake from the heat and cook the next batch. Makes four pancakes.
6. Top with the blueberries to serve.

Pineapple Kale Smoothie

This smoothie is packed with proteins, vitamins, and minerals to give you energy to perform your best throughout the day. Its anti inflammatory properties suppress pro inflammatory indicators like cytokines.

Nutritional Information

Cholesterol	3mg
Dietary Fiber	4g
Sodium	149mg
Protein	8g
Sugars	13g
Total Carbohydrates	527g
Total Fat	9g
Calories per serving	187

Time: 5 minutes

Serving Size: 2

Ingredients:

- ¼ cup of diced pineapple pieces
- 2 cups of chopped kale with stalks removed
- 1 cup of soymilk
- 1 cup of sliced banana pieces
- 2 tablespoons of peanut butter
- 1 cup of ice cubes

Directions:

1. Blend all ingredients in a blender until smooth and creamy and serve immediately.

Energizing Chia Pounding

Chia seeds are packed with fiber, antioxidants, and protein, to give you energy for a productive day. They also contain omega-3 fatty acids to help fight inflammation.

Nutritional Information

Calcium	54 mg
Dietary Fiber	2 g
Iron	4.9 mg
Vitamin A	155 mg
Potassium	79 mg
Sodium	123 mg
Protein	13 g
Total Carbohydrates	13 g
Total Fat	16 g
Calories per serving	258

Time: 2 hours

Serving Size: 1

Ingredients:

- 2 tablespoons of chia seeds
- ¼ cup of cooked quinoa
- Dash of stevia
- A pinch of cinnamon
- ¾ cup of cashew milk

- ¼ teaspoon vanilla protein powder

Directions:

1. Combine all the ingredients in a jar and mix well.
2. Cover the jar tightly and refrigerate for two or more hours.

3. Serve with any toppings you desire such as fresh berries.

Nutty Chocolate Smoothie Bowl

This is a gluten-free, vegan recipe perfect for chocolate lovers. This recipe contains peanut butter, which is a source of healthy fats.

Nutritional Information

Calcium	138mg
Dietary Fiber	12g
Iron	2.6g
Potassium	1416mg
Sodium	260mg
Vitamin A	150IU
Vitamin C	25.7mg
Protein	6.5g
Sugars	39g
Total Carbohydrates	79g
Total Fat	19g
Calories per serving	485

Time: 5 minutes

Serving Size: 2

Ingredients:

- 4 bananas
- 1 cup of ice cubes
- ⅔ cup of almond milk
- 4 tablespoons of peanut butter
- 4 tablespoons of dark cacao powder
- 2 tablespoons of chia seeds

For Topping

- 1 sliced banana
- 1 tablespoon of dark chocolate chips
- 1 tablespoon of peanut butter to drizzle

Directions:

1. Combine all the smoothie ingredients and blend in a blender until a smooth consistency is reached.
2. Microwave one tablespoon of peanut butter in a small bowl for 30 seconds.
3. Transfer the smoothie to two bowls and top with the topping.

Cinnamon Quinoa Breakfast

Quinoa is packed with protein, gluten-free, high in several essential nutrients like fiber, calcium, and potassium, has antioxidants, and is anti inflammatory.

Nutritional Information

Calcium	363mg
Dietary Fiber	8.2g
Iron	5g
Potassium	678mg
Sodium	185mg
Vitamin D	1mcg
Protein	13.1g
Sugars	0.1g
Total Carbohydrates	59.4g
Total Fat	8.7g
Calories per serving	359

Time: 35 minutes

Serving Size: 1

Ingredients:

- 1/2 cup of rinsed quinoa

- 1 cup of unsweetened almond milk
- 1 chai tea bag
- 1 teaspoon of cinnamon

Directions:

1. Bring the milk, quinoa, and chai tea bag to a boil in a small saucepan under medium heat. Once the mixture has started boiling, remove the tea bag.
2. Reduce the heat to low, cover the pan, and cook for 15 -20 minutes
3. Remove from the heat and keep covered for 10 more minutes so that the almond milk can be absorbed.
4. Serve by sprinkling cinnamon on top.

Savory Chickpea Pancakes

Vegan and packed with fiber and protein, chickpeas improve insulin resistance and reduce inflammatory indicators.

Nutritional Information

Calcium	363mg
Calcium	203mg
Dietary Fiber	25.9g
Iron	8g
Potassium	1626mg
Sodium	81mg
Protein	13.1g
Sugars	13.5g
Total Carbohydrates	81.7g
Total Fat	28.1g
Calories per serving	643

Time: 35 minutes

Serving Size: 1

Ingredients:

- ¼ cup of chopped green onion
- ¼ cup of finely chopped red bell pepper
- ½ cup of chickpea flour

- ¼ teaspoon of garlic powder
- ¼ teaspoon of baking powder
- ⅔ of cup water
- ½ avocado
- Salt and black pepper to taste

Directions:

1. Whisk together the chickpea flour, garlic powder, salt, pepper, and baking powder.
2. Add water and whisk until there are no lumps and to create air bubbles, which make the pancakes fluffy. Stir in the onion and bell peppers.
3. In a large skillet that has been sprayed with nonstick spray, over medium heat, pour in the batter to make one large pancake. Cook for five minutes on each side or until each side is golden brown and the pancake does not fall apart.
4. Serve with sliced avocado on top.

Vanilla Smoothie Bowl

Vanilla contains a compound called vanillin, which is anti cancer, anti tumor, and fights inflammation by decreasing the production of proinflammatory indication such as cytokines.

Nutritional Information

Dietary Fiber	13.7g
Sodium	327mg
Protein	11.5g
Sugars	10.6g
Total Carbohydrates	42.9g
Total Fat	22.5g
Calories per serving	419

Time: 25 minutes

Serving Size: 1

Ingredients:

- 3 ripe sliced bananas
- ½ cup of ice cubes
- ½ ripe avocado
- ¼ cup of unsweetened almond milk
- 1 scoop of vanilla protein powder
- ½ teaspoon of raw spirulina powder
- Chia seeds for topping

Directions:

1. Blend all the smoothie ingredients in a blender until smooth, creamy consistency has been reached.
2. Transfer to a bowl and top with chia seeds.

Lunch Recipes

Balsamic Avocado Tomato Toast

Avocados lower the levels of proinflammatory indications and contain compounds that reduce cancer risk. Tomatoes are high in vitamin C, potassium, and lycopene — an antioxidant that is anti inflammatory.

Nutritional Information

Calcium	122mg
Dietary Fiber	13.7g
Iron	4mg
Potassium	1520mg
Sodium	293mg
Protein	13.7g
Sugars	8.8g
Total Carbohydrates	51.2g
Total Fat	46.6g
Calories per serving	669

Time: 25 minutes

Serving Size: 1

Ingredients:

- 2 slices of multigrain bread
- 1 teaspoon of olive oil - 6 thin slices of tomatoes
- ½ cup of mashed ripe avocado
- ½ cup of balsamic vinegar
- ¼ cup of chopped basil
- Salt and black pepper to taste

Directions:

1. Create a balsamic reduction by boiling the balsamic vinegar over medium heat and whisking constantly.
2. Reduce the heat to low and simmer for 12 minutes or until the liquid has been reduced to a thick consistency. Test the consistency with a spoon.
3. Toast each piece of bread then drizzle with olive oil.
4. Evenly coat the toast with the mashed avocado then layer the tomatoes on top.
5. Drizzle with the balsamic reduction then garnish with chopped basil, salt, and pepper.
6. Serve immediately.

Vegan BLT Wraps

Tempeh is a soy product and will be the bacon substitute for this delicious wrap. This item is a close relative of tofu but is firmer in texture. It has a mild flavor so you can dress it up or down as you desire.

Nutritional Information

Dietary Fiber	3.7g
Sodium	722mg
Protein	23g
Sugars	4.1g
Total Carbohydrates	20.5g
Total Fat	26g
Calories per serving	382

Time: 15 minutes

Serving Size: 2

Ingredients:

- ½ package of ⅛" tempeh
- 4 washed and dried large leaves of green lettuce
- ½ teaspoon of olive oil
- 1 ½ tablespoon of soy sauce
- 1 ½ maple syrup
- ¼ teaspoon onion powder
- ⅛ teaspoon of cumin
- 4 slices of avocado
- 4 slices of tomato

- 1 tablespoon of vegan mayonnaise
- Black pepper to taste

Directions:

1. Add soy sauce, maple syrup, onion powder, cumin, and black powder in a medium bowl and whisk to make a marinade.
2. Add tempeh slices to the marinade and allow to soak for a few minutes.
3. Cut the bottom of the lettuce leaves into an inverted V shape to make the folding process easier.
4. Heat the olive oil in a large skillet over medium heat. Sear the tempeh on each side for three to four minutes. The edges will become blackened slightly.
5. To assemble the wraps, layer two lettuce leaves so that the bottom parts overlap in the center about three inches. Arrange the tempeh, tomato, avocado, and mayonnaise in the leaves.
6. To fold the wrap, tuck in the ends, and roll lengthwise. Cut this into two pieces and plate.
7. Repeat with the other two lettuce leaves.
8. Serve.

Quick Chicken Salad

This recipe contains grapes, which is an antioxidants, namely flavonoids and resveratrol, both of which have anti inflammatory properties.

Nutritional Information

Calcium	63mg
Dietary Fiber	9.1
Iron	4mg
Potassium	1248mg
Sodium	1268mg
Protein	38.7g
Sugars	25.9g
Total Carbohydrates	48.2g
Total Fat	50.3g
Calories per serving	772

Time: 10 minutes

Serving Size: 2

Ingredients:

- 1 ½ cup skinless chicken breast (cooked and shredded)
- 2 cups of halved red grapes
- ¼ cup of chopped red onion
- 1 diced avocado

- ½ cup of cashew nuts

For Vinaigrette

- ⅛ teaspoon salt
- ½ tablespoon balsamic vinegar
- 1 tablespoon olive oil

Directions:

1. Toss the salad ingredients in a large bowl.
2. Make the salad dressing by combining the Vinaigrette ingredients.
3. Drizzle vinaigrette over salad and toss until the salad ingredients are thoroughly coated.
4. Serve

Quinoa Veggie Bowl

Bell peppers are loaded with vitamin C and antioxidants like quercetin that fight chronic inflammation.

Nutritional Information

Calcium	19mg
Dietary Fiber	2.6g
Iron	2mg
Sodium	4mg
Potassium	235mg
Protein	4.4g
Sugars	1.4g
Total Carbohydrates	20.5g
Total Fat	10.2g
Calories per serving	187

Time: 45 minutes

Serving Size: 6 (1 ½ cup per serving)

Ingredients:

- 1 cup washed quinoa
- ½ cups of water
- 1 cup of chopped green bell pepper
- 1 cup of chopped red bell pepper
- ¼ cup of olive oil
- 2 tablespoons of apple cider vinegar

- 2 tablespoons of chopped parsley
- Salt and pepper to taste

Directions:

1. Light toast the quinoa in a medium saucepan over medium heat to remove any remaining liquid and to add a nutty flavor.
2. Add water and bring to a boil. Reduce heat and allow the quinoa to simmer for 10 minutes or until the quinoa is fluffy.
3. While the quinoa simmers, make the salad dressing by mixing the olive oil, apple cider vinegar, salt, and pepper.
4. Remove the quinoa from heat and chill in the refrigerator for a few minutes.
5. Add the peppers.
6. Pour the salad dressing over the quinoa mixture and toss with a fork.
7. Serve.

Tomato Cucumber Toast

In addition to being hydrating, anti cancerous, and alkalizing, cucumbers contain flavonoids, which are anti inflammatory antioxidants.

Nutritional Information

Protein	3g
Sugars	4g
Total Carbohydrates	24g
Total Fat	8g
Calories per serving	177

Time: 45 minutes

Serving Size: 6 (1 ½ cup per serving)

Ingredients:

- 1 small diced tomato
- 1 diced cucumber
- 1 teaspoon of olive oil
- A pinch of dried oregano
- 2 teaspoons of vegan mayonnaise
- 2 slices of whole grain bread
- 1 teaspoon of balsamic glaze
- Salt and black pepper to taste

Directions:

1. Combine the vegetables with olive oil and oregano in a medium bowl.
2. Add the salt and pepper and toss.

3. Smear one side of the bread sliced with the mayonnaise.
4. Top with the veggie mixture and balsamic glaze.

Simple Lemon Tuna Salad

Lemons help improve digestion, enhance liver function, and fight acidity and inflammation in the stomach.

Nutritional Information

Calcium	12mg
Cholesterol	55mg
Dietary Fiber	0.8g
Iron	2mg
Potassium	735mg
Protein g	48.1g
Sugars	0.8
Total Carbohydrates	3.2g
Total Fat	30.7g
Calories per serving	484

Time: 10 minutes

Serving Size: 1

Ingredients:

- ⅓ cup of diced cucumber
- ½ cup of small avocado
- 1 teaspoon of lemon juice
- 1 can of 6 oz f tuna
- 1 tablespoon olive oil
- 2 leaves of romaine lettuce

- Salt and black pepper to taste

Directions:

1. Combine the cucumber, avocado, and lemon juice in a medium bowl.
2. Open a can of tuna, drain and dump into a small bowl. Flake with a fork and mix with the olive oil.
3. Add the tuna mixture to the avocado and cucumber mixture.
4. Place the tuna salad on top of the lettuce leaves.
5. Sprinkle with salt and pepper to taste.
6. Serve.

Paleo Veggie Delight Pizza

One ingredient in this recipe is mushroom and these contain several anti inflammatory components such as indolic compounds, vitamins and fatty acids. Mushrooms also contain antioxidants and anticancer components.

Nutritional Information

Calcium	147mg
Cholesterol	amg
Dietary Fiber	6.9g
Iron	4mg
Sodium	1322mg
Potassium	1639mg
Vitamin D	5mcg
Protein	26.5g
Sugars	13.4
Total Carbohydrates	26g
Total Fat	22.6g
Calories per serving	388

Time: 45 minutes

Serving Size: 4

Ingredients:

- 2 ½ cup of soy flour, plus more for dusting
- 1/2 teaspoon baking powder
- 1 teaspoon Italian seasoning
- ⅛ teaspoon of garlic powder
- ½ teaspoon of salt
- 3 teaspoons of baking soda
- 3 teaspoons of white vinegar
- 5 tablespoons of olive oil
- ½ cup of chopped red tomatoes
- ¼ cup sliced red onion
- ½ cup of sliced green bell pepper
- ¼ cup of sliced black olives
- 2 sliced cremini mushrooms

Directions:

1. Preheat your oven to 425 degrees F.
2. Prepare a baking sheet by brushing it with olive oil and dusting it with flour so that the entire surface is coated.
3. In a bowl, beginning making the dough by hisking in sieved soy flour, baking powder, Italian seasoning, garlic powder, and salt.
4. In a small bowl, mix the baking soda and white vinegar to make an egg substitute. Add this to the flour mixture along with the olive oil. Stir to form a dough. If the dough is too dry, add water a teaspoon at a time until the dough is soft and malleable.
5. Roll out the dough to a quarter of an inch thickness.
6. Transfer the dough to the baking sheet.
7. Bake for 10 minutes or until crust is golden brown.
8. Top with the remaining ingredients and bake for five minutes.
9. Slice and serve.

Dinner Recipes

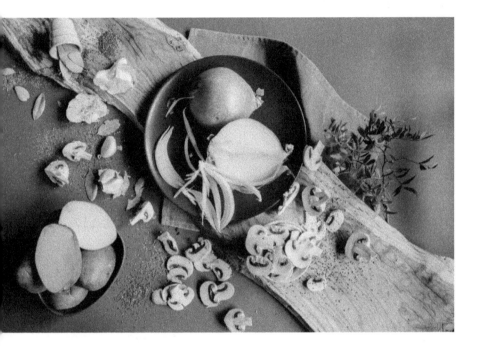

Hearty Lentil Kale Soup

Lentils are high in fiber and magnesium. Magnesium helps reduce chronic inflammation.

Nutritional Information

Calcium	89mg
Dietary Fiber	12g
Iron	3mg
Sodium	170mg
Potassium	345mg
Protein	11g
Sugars	4g
Total Carbohydrates	29g
Total Fat	5g
Calories per serving	200

Time: 45 minutes

Serving Size: 6 (1 ½ cup per serving)

Ingredients:

- 2 tablespoons of olive oil
- 1 cup of chopped yellow onion
- 1 cup of diced carrot
- 2 teaspoons of peeled and minced garlic
- 1 cup of rinsed brown lentils
- 4 cups of water

- 1 ½ cup of vegetable stock
- 1 tablespoon of dried basil
- 2 large chopped tomatoes
- 1 bunch of kale - 1 teaspoon of salt
- ⅛ teaspoon of ground black pepper

Directions:

1. Heat the oil in a large pot over medium heat. Saute the onions, carrots, and garlic for five minutes.
2. Add water and bring to a boil.
3. Add the lentils and simmer for 20 minutes.
4. Add the stock, basil and tomatoes. Cover the pot and cook for no more than 10 minutes.
5. Add remaining ingredients. Reduce to low heat, cover and simmer for three more minutes.

Baked Chicken Veggie Dinner

A protein in chicken called hydrolysates has many anti inflammatory effects. This making chicken a great addition to the anti inflammation diet as long as it is consumed in moderation that it. Squash is high in fiber and has been scientifically proven to lower the levels of inflammation indicators in the body.

Nutritional Information

Calcium	89mg
Dietary Fiber	8g
Iron	3mg
Sodium	680mg
Potassium	1135mg
Protein	22g
Sugars	7g
Cholesterol	80mg
Total Carbohydrates	30g
Total Fat	18g
Calories per serving	348

Time: 1 hour

Serving Size: 4

Ingredients:

- 1 pound trimmed and halved Brussels sprouts
- 1 pound diced butternut squash
- ½ cup of yellow onion
- 1 thinly sliced lemon
- Lemon juice
- 3 large minced garlic cloves
- 4 tablespoons of olive oil
- 2 tablespoons of balsamic vinegar
- 1 tablespoon of apple cider vinegar
- 1 ½ teaspoon of salt
- 1/2 teaspoon black pepper
- 1 teaspoon of ground pepper
- A pinch of freshly grated nutmeg
- 4 bone-in chicken thighs
- 1 teaspoon of fennel seeds
- 1 teaspoon of crushed red pepper
- 1 teaspoon of ground paprika
- 1 teaspoon of garlic powder
- 4 chopped fresh sage leaves

Directions:

1. Preheat your oven to 450 degrees F.
2. In a large bowl toss the Brussels sprouts, squash, onion, lemon, garlic, two tablespoons of olive oil, balsamic vinegar, one teaspoon of salt, black pepper and nutmeg. Spread the coated veggies on a large baking sheet.
3. Make the marinade for the chicken by combining the remaining oil and salt, apple cider vinegar, red pepper, fennel seeds, sage, paprika, and garlic powder. Coat the chicken in this marinade and evenly arrange the chicken on top of the veggies.
4. Bake this for 35 minutes or until the chicken and veggies are cooked all the way through. Your can check to see if it is fully cooked by inserting the sharp tip of the knife through the chicken and veggies. If

clear liquid runs from the chicken, it is done. If the knife goes through the veggies easily, they are done.

5. Plate the chicken and veggies and squeeze lemon juice on top to serve.

Baked Cod and Chickpea Salad

This is a Mediterranean recipe. Cod contains an anti inflammatory agent called carotenoid, which gives the fish its pink color.

Nutritional Information

Dietary Fiber	8g
Sodium	445mg
Protein	35g
Sugars	7g
Cholesterol	69mg
Total Carbohydrates	33g
Total Fat	10g
Calories per serving	363

Time: 45 minutes

Serving Size: 4

Ingredients:

- 4 5-ounce skinless, boneless cod fillets
- 2 cups of spinach
- 1 teaspoon of olive oil
- ½ cup of pitted and minced olives
- 2 minced cloves of garlic
- 2 tablespoons of lemon juice
- ½ teaspoon of lemon zest
- ⅛ teaspoon of salt

- ¼ teaspoon of ground black pepper
- 2 red bell pepper

For the Chickpea Salad

- 2 cups of cooked chickpeas
- 2 teaspoons of olive oil
- ½ cup of chopped red onion
- 1 minced garlic clove
- ½ cup of minced parsley
- 10 pitted and chopped olives
- 1 tablespoon dried oregano
- ¼ cup of lemon juice
- 1 ½ teaspoon lemon zest
- ¼ cup of ground black pepper
- 1 ½ cup of chopped tomatoes

Directions:

1. Preheat your oven to 350 degrees F.
2. Combine the minced olives, salt and pepper, lemon juice, and garlic in a small bowl. Set aside.
3. Trim, half and de-seed the bell peppers. Arrange the peppers on a prepared baking sheet skin side down. Brush the tops with a quarter teaspoon of olive oil. Top with the spinach and cod.
4. Add the remaining olive oil to the olive mixture and spread evenly over the cod.
5. Bake this for 23 minutes.
6. To make the chickpea salad, heat the olive oil in a medium skillet over medium heat. Saute the onion and garlic for one minute.
7. Add the chickpeas, a quarter cup parsley, lemon juice, oregano and one tablespoon of water. Cook for five minutes and stir often.
8. Add the olives and tomatoes. Cook and stir until all the liquid evaporates. This should be less than ten minutes.

9. Stir in the remaining parsley, lemon zest, and black pepper. Remove the salad from the heat.
10. Plate the cod mixture and serve with chickpea salad.

Rosemary Salmon Dinner

This recipes feature yellow mustard, which is a blend of mustard seeds, turmeric, salt, white vinegar and spices. As a result of it compounds, namely turmeric, it has powerful anti inflammatory properties

Nutritional Information

Calcium	56mg
Cholesterol	50mg
Dietary Fiber	0.4g
Iron	1mg
Sodium	66mg
Potassium	475mg
Protein	22.3g
Sugars	1.6g
Cholesterol	50mg
Total Carbohydrates	2.3g
Total Fat	7.2g
Calories per serving	159

Time: 40 minutes

Serving Size: 4

Ingredients:

- 4 4-oz salmon fillets
- 1 tablespoon yellow mustard
- 2 minced cloves garlic
- 1 tablespoon chopped green onions
- 2 teaspoon of chopped thyme leaves, plus more branches for garnish
- 2 teaspoons of chopped rosemary
- ½ teaspoon of lemon juice
- Lemon slices for garnish
- Salt and black pepper to taste

Directions:

1. Prepare your broiler.
2. Prepare a baking sheet with parchment paper.
3. To make seasoning mixture, combine all the ingredients except for the salmon and garnish ingredients.
4. Place the salmon fillets on a baking sheet and spread the seasoning mixture over the fish.
5. Broil for seven minutes.
6. Plate and serve by garnishing with the lemon slices and thyme.

Creamy Tomato Soup

Black pepper, an ingredient in this recipe, fights inflammation with the active compound called piperine.

Nutritional Information

Calcium	35mg
Dietary Fiber	1.2g
Iron	3mg
Sodium	526mg
Potassium	527mg
Protein	44.9g
Sugars	1.9g
Cholesterol	135mg
Total Carbohydrates	3.1g
Total Fat	12.2g
Calories per serving	424

Time: 30 minutes

Serving Size: 6

Ingredients:

- 4 roasted mashed tomatoes
- 1 cup of water
- 1/4 teaspoon of black pepper
- 1 teaspoon of salt

- 1/3 cup fresh basil
- 2 tablespoons olive oil
- 2 pounds boneless skinless chicken thighs, cute into 1 -inch chunks
- 1 cup of coconut milk

Directions:

1. In a cast-iron pan, add the tomato, water, salt, pepper, basil, and olive oil. Bring to a boil over medium heat, stirring occasionally.
2. Add the chicken and cook for 25 minutes.
3. Remove from the heat and blend the soup in the immersion blend.
4. Add the mixture back to the pan once a smooth consistency has been reached.
5. Add the coconut milk and stir to thoroughly combine.
6. Cook on low heat for five more minutes.
7. Serve warm.

Brown Rice Bowl with Roasted Red Pepper Sauce

Brown rice is an unrefined grain item that helps fight inflammation and is high in fiber.

Nutritional Information

Calcium	75mg
Cholesterol	1mg
Dietary Fiber	4.2g
Iron	3mg
Sodium	80mg
Potassium	404mg
Protein	6.8g
Sugars	1.6g
Cholesterol	1mg
Total Carbohydrates	23g
Total Fat	8.5g
Calories per serving	187

Time: 30 minutes

Serving Size: 1

Ingredients:

- 1 cup of cooked brown rice

- ½ cup of spinach
- ½ cup of diced cucumber
- ¼ cup of cooked white beans
- 4 pitted olives
- ¼ cup of thinly sliced red onion
- 1 tablespoon of thinly chopped parsley
- 1 teaspoon of olive oil,
- ½ teaspoon of lemon juice
- Salt and black pepper to taste

For Roasted Red Pepper Sauce

- 1 roasted red bell pepper
- 1 minced clove garlic
- 1/2 teaspoon salt
- ½ tablespoon juice lemon
- 1/2 cup olive oil
- 1/2 cup almonds

Directions:

1. To make the roasted red pepper sauce, pulse all the ingredients in a blender or food processor to a thick consistency.
2. Build your brown rice bowl, but layer all ingredients on top of the brown rice.
3. Pour roasted red pepper sauce on top and serve.

Cauliflower Roast

Cauliflower helps the body get rid of waste because it contains sulphur. It also contains the compound 3-carbinol, which helps inflammation.

Nutritional Information

Calcium	68mg
Dietary Fiber	6.7g
Iron	2mg
Sodium	74mg
Potassium	884mg
Protein	5.4g
Sugars	7.3g
Total Carbohydrates	16g
Total Fat	5.1g
Calories per serving	115

Time: 1 hour, 20 minutes

Serving Size: 4

Ingredients:

- 2 pounds of cauliflower
- 1 1/2 cup of cherry tomatoes
- 4 minced cloves garlic
- 4 teaspoon of olive oil
- 1/4 teaspoon of crushed red pepper flakes

- 1/8 teaspoon of paprika
- 1/4 cup of chopped parsley
- Salt and black pepper to taste

Directions:

1. Preheat your oven to 400 degrees F.
2. Toss the tomatoes with three tablespoons of olive oil, salt, black pepper, garlic, and red pepper flakes.
3. Place this mixture in a baking tray.
4. Trim the large green leaves and stems from the cauliflower. Sit the cauliflower flat in the center of the tomatoes. Drizzle it with the remaining olive oil and sprinkle with salt and pepper.
5. Roast for an hour. The cauliflower is done when it is easily pierced with a sharp knife.
6. Remove the tray from the oven and sprinkle with parsley.
7. Cut the cauliflower into wedges and serve with a side of tomatoes.

Chapter 5: Week 2 Recipes

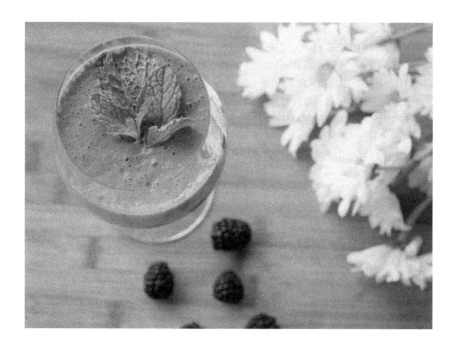

Breakfast Recipes

Coconut Strawberry Smoothie

Get a boost of fiber and protein with this recipe. This is especially great to power you through a morning workout.

Nutritional Information

Dietary Fiber	8g
Protein	21g
Sugars	22g
Total Carbohydrates	31g
Total Fat	7g
Calories per serving	270

Time: 10 minutes

Serving Size: 1

Ingredients:

- 1 cup of sliced strawberries
- 1 cup of coconut milk
- 1 cup of ice cubes
- ¼ cup of vanilla protein powder
- 2 teaspoons of maple syrup
- 1 teaspoon of vanilla extract
- 1 teaspoon of ground flaxseeds

Directions:

1. Blend all ingredients in a blender until a smooth consistency is reached.
2. Serve.

Beet Berry Smoothie Bowl

Beets are great for boosting the immune system to lessen the likelihood of triggering inflammation. They also purify the blood and increase energy. And the best part, they help this smoothie taste divine.

Nutritional Information

Calcium	329mg
Cholesterol	135mg
Dietary Fiber	14.3g
Iron	4mg
Potassium	1186mg
Vitamin D	1mcg
Protein	35.8g
Sugars	28.5g
Total Carbohydrates	58.7g
Total Fat	10.1g
Calories per serving	464

Time: 10 minutes

Serving Size: 1

Ingredients:

- 3/4 cup chopped roasted beets
- 3/4 cup raspberries

- ¼ cup ice cubes
- 1/2 cup unsweetened Almond milk
- 1 tablespoon lime juice
- 1 scoop vanilla protein powder
- 1 tablespoon flax seeds
- 1 ripe banana

Directions:

1. Blend all ingredients in a blender until a smooth consistency is reached.
2. Serve.

Coconut Almond Toast With Dark Chocolate

The almond chocolate butter give Nutella a run for its money. The nutritional value is great too. Coconuts have several benefits such as being antimicrobial, analgesic, and antipyretic in addition to being anti inflammatory.

Nutritional Information

Calcium	62mg
Dietary Fiber	3.9g
Iron	2mg
Potassium	92mg
Protein	6.4g
Sugars	5.4g
Total Carbohydrates	18g
Total Fat	3g
Calories per serving	180

Time: 50 minutes

Serving Size: 2

Ingredients:

- 2 slice of whole wheat bread
- 2 tablespoons of coconut flakes
- Roasted almonds
- A pinch of salt

For Almond Chocolate Butter

- 2 cups of unsalted roasted almonds
- 1/4 teaspoon of vanilla extract
- 1/3 cup of dark chocolate chips
- 1 teaspoon of coconut oil
- 2 tablespoons of dark cocoa powder
- 1 teaspoon of maple syrup
- 1 teaspoon of salt

Directions:

1. To make the almond chocolate butter, start by pulsing the almonds in a food processor for about 12 minutes. Scrap the sides down when the almonds stick to it. Allow the almonds to reach a creamy consistency.
2. In a small pan over the lowest heat setting, melt the chocolate chips and coconut oil, stirring until smooth.
3. Add the melted chocolate and the rest of the ingredients to the almond butter and process against for two minutes.
4. Transfer the mixture to an airtight container and store at room temperature or in the refrigerator, using as needed.
5. To make the toast, spread the almond chocolate butter on one side of each piece of bread.
6. Top with the coconut flakes and almonds and sprinkle some salt.

Tofu Egg Breakfast Sandwich

Tofu is a soy-based product and is rich in antioxidants and omega-3 fatty acids, both of which are anti inflammatory.

Nutritional Information

Calcium	488mg
Dietary Fiber	7.3g
Iron	8mg
Potassium	1387mg
Protein	52.2g
Sugars	9.4g
Total Carbohydrates	45.9g
Total Fat	46.3g
Calories per serving	757

Time: 45 minutes

Serving Size: 2

Ingredients:

For "Egg"

- 2 slabs of tofu
- 1/4 tsp turmeric
- olive oil
- Salt and pepper to taste

For Strawberry Jam

- 2 cups of de-stemmed and chopped strawberries
- 2 tablespoons of maple syrup
- water
- 2 tablespoons of chia seed.

Other Ingredients

- 2 multigrain buns
- ½ avocado, mashed
- 3 slices of tomato
- 4 slices of prepared tempeh (See Veggie BLT Wraps recipe)

Directions:

1. To make the strawberry jam, blend the strawberry, chia seeds, and maple syrup for one minute. Add water a tablespoon at a time until you reach your preferred consistency.
2. Pour mixture into a small saucepan and bring to a boil over medium heat. Simmer for six minutes or until the jam thickens.
3. Remove from the heat and pour into a heat resistant airtight container. Allow the jam to cool then refrigerate for up to a week, using as needed.
4. To prepare the eggy tofu, blot each slice with a paper towel to remove any excess liquid. Sprinkle the tofu with turmeric and salt and pepper on both sides.
5. Heat the olive oil in a medium skillet over medium heat and add the tofu. Cover the pan and cook for two minutes.
6. Flip the tofu and cook until the edges start to brown and tofu is fluffy.
7. To assemble the sandwich, slice your bread in half and toast it. Spread jam on one side of each half. Add the mashed avocado to the other halves. Layer the tofu slices on the jam side. continue building the sandwich by adding tomatoes and tempeh

slices.Close the sandwich with the other half and serve.

Vegan French Toast

This recipe contains nutritional yeast, which supports a healthy immune system and helps reduce inflammation caused by bacterial infection.

Nutritional Information

Calcium	150mg
Dietary Fiber	13.6g
Iron	7mg
Potassium	984mg
Protein	17.3g
Sugars	26.3g
Total Carbohydrates	72.9g
Total Fat	45.9g
Calories per serving	738

Time: 20 minutes

Serving Size: 1

Ingredients:

- 2 slices of whole wheat bread
- 1/2 cup of almond milk
- 1 tablespoon of maple syrup
- 2 tablespoons of whole wheat flour
- 1 tablespoon of nutritional yeast
- 1 teaspoon of cinnamon

- ¼ teaspoon of ground nutmeg
- A pinch of salt
- Coconut oil

Toppings

- Maple syrup
- Strawberry slices

Directions:

1. Whisk together all the ingredients except for the bread and coconut oil.
2. Place the bread in a shallow bowl and pour the wet mixture over it. Ensure that the bread slices soak up the wet mixture.
3. Heat the coconut oil in a large skillet over medium heat. Add the bread slices and cook both sides until they are golden brown.
4. Serve warm with the toppings.

Homemade Blueberry Waffles

Packed with antioxidants and phytoflavinoids, blackberries are high in potassium and vitamins, properties that lower the risk of heart disease, cancer, and inflammation.

Nutritional Information

Calcium	170mg
Dietary Fiber	8.5g
Iron	8mg
Potassium	755mg
Protein	16.8g
Sugars	19g
Total Carbohydrates	122.7g
Total Fat	21g
Calories per serving	811

Time: 20 minutes

Serving Size: 2

Ingredients:

- ¾ cups almond milk
- 3/4 tablespoons apple cider vinegar
- 1 tablespoon of melted coconut oil
- 2 tablespoons maple syrup
- ¼ teaspoon vanilla extract
- 2 cups of wheat flour

- 1 teaspoon of baking powder
- 2 tablespoons of flax meal (Flax seeds pulsed into a powder)
- ¼ teaspoon cinnamon
- A pinch of salt
- ½ cup of quartered blueberries
- Maple syrup for topping

Directions:

1. Preheat your waffle iron.
2. Mix the dry ingredients in a large bowl.
3. Mix the wet ingredients in another bowl.
4. Add wet ingredients to dry and mix until they are all just combined. Do not over mix.
5. Scoop the batter into your waffle iron and follow the cooking instructions of your waffle iron. Place the blueberries pieces on the top of the waffle mixture before pressing the iron.
6. Serve the waffle hot, topped with the maple syrup. These waffles can be stored in the freezer and popped into the toaster when needed.

Maple Coconut Oats

Maple syrup has a compound that has been scientifically proven to prevent inflammation. It is called quebecol.

Nutritional Information

Calcium	40mg
Dietary Fiber	23.1g
Iron	31mg
Potassium	1128mg
Protein	12.5g
Sugars	19.4g
Total Carbohydrates	50.4g
Total Fat	98.2g
Calories per serving	1071

Time: 20 minutes

Serving Size: 2

Ingredients:

- 1/3 cup of rolled oats
- 1 teaspoon of maple syrup
- 1 cup of coconut milk

Toppings

- Coconut flakes
- 1 tablespoon of crushed walnuts

- ¼ cup of blackberries

Directions:

1. Add the oats, maple syrup, and coconut milk to a small saucepan over medium heat.
2. Reduce the heat and cook the oats until the mixture as thickened, stirring constantly.
3. Pour the oats into a bowl and serve warm with toppings.

Lunch Recipes

Curry Apple Tuna Salad

Apples are high in antioxidants that help fight inflammation.

Nutritional Information

Calcium	13mg
Dietary Fiber	1g
Iron	1mg
Potassium	436mg
Protein	30.3g
Sugars	2.9g
Total Carbohydrates	5.1g
Total Fat	11.9g
Calories per serving	255

Time: 20 minutes

Serving Size: 4

Ingredients:

- 1 pound of tuna
- ½ cup of diced green apples
- ¼ cup of chopped parsley

- 1/3 cups of vegan mayo
- 1 teaspoon of curry powder
- 1 teaspoon of salt
- ½ teaspoon of lime juice

Directions:

1. To keep the apple slices from turning brown, combine the lime juice with 1 cup of water and place the piece in the water.
2. When it is time to assemble your salad, drain the apple pieces. Add all the ingredients to a medium bowl. Mix well.
3. Serve and chill any remainder.

Broccoli Tempeh Salad

Broccoli is rich in antioxidant that deduce the levels of proinflammatory indicators like cytokines.

Nutritional Information

Calcium	176mg
Dietary Fiber	4.8g
Iron	3mg
Potassium	854mg
Protein	23g
Sugars	4.3g
Total Carbohydrates	24.2g
Total Fat	24.6g
Calories per serving	386

Time: 25 minutes

Serving Size: 4

Ingredients:

- 4 cooked and diced tempeh slices (See the Vegan BLT Wrap recipe for directions)
- 3 heads broccoli
- 2 carrots
- 1/2 red onion
- 1/2 cup of dried cranberries
- 1/2 cup of sliced almonds

- A pinch of salt

For Salad Dressing

- 1/2 cup of vegan mayonnaise
- 3 tablespoons of apple cider vinegar
- Salt and black pepper to taste

Directions:

1. Prepare the vegetables by cutting the broccoli into bite-size pieces, shredding the carrots and thinly slicing the red onion.
2. Bring four cups of water to a boil. Add a pinch of salt and add the broccoli pieces. Cook for a minute and a half.
3. Prepare an ice bath by adding ice cubes to a bowl of water.
4. Use a slotted spoon to place the cooked broccoli pieces into the ice bath. When the pieces have become cooled, use a colander to drain.
5. In a large bowl, add the rest of the salad ingredients.
6. To make the salad dressing, whisk together all the ingredients.
7. Pour the dressing over the broccoli mistires and gentle fold to incorporate all the ingredients.
8. Plate and serve.

Loaded Veggie Sandwich

Bean sprouts, an ingredient in this recipe, contain antioxidants that lower CRP levels.

Nutritional Information

Calcium	53mg
Dietary Fiber	2.3g
Iron	1mg
Potassium	299mg
Protein	3.7g
Sugars	5.3g
Total Carbohydrates	16.9g
Total Fat	3.4g
Calories per serving	106

Time: 25 minutes

Serving Size: 4

Ingredients:

- 2 slices whole wheat bread
- 3 tablespoons vegan mayonnaise
- 1 teaspoon of yellow mustard
- 1 lettuce leaf
- 1/4 cup bean sprouts
- 2 slices of tomato
- 2 slices of cucumber

- Thin slices of red onion

Directions:

1. Toast the bread.
2. Spread mayonnaise on one side of one slice and mustard on one side of the other slice of bread,
3. Layer on the vegetables on the mayonnaise side of that slice of bread.
4. Place the other slice of bread mustard-side down on this.
5. Slice diagonally and serve.

Veggie Burger with Jalapeno Mayo

Sweet, spicy, tangy, and good for you, this veggie burger is hearty enough to fuel the rest of your day and flavorful enough to have your tastebuds singing. It is packed with anti inflammation ingredients that are easy on your gut.

Nutritional Information

Calcium	235mg
Dietary Fiber	14.4g
Iron	7mg
Sodium	447mg
Potassium	1472mg
Protein	25.3g
Sugars	9.8g
Total Carbohydrates	87.6g
Total Fat	22.2g
Calories per serving	628

Time: 45 minutes

Serving Size: 6

Ingredients:

For Patty

- 1 cup of cooked brown rice
- 1 cup of raw walnuts

- 1/2 tablespoon olive oil plus extra
- ¾ cups of finely chopped white onion
- 1 tablespoon of chili powder,
- 1 tablespoon of cumin powder
- 1 tablespoon of paprika
- 1/2 tsp each salt
- ½ teaspoon of black pepper
- 1 1/2 cups cooked black beans
- 1/3 cup panko bread crumbs
- 3 tablespoons vegan BBQ sauce

Jalapeno Mayo

- 6 tablespoons of vegan mayonnaise
- 4teaspoon dried jalapeno
- 3 tablespoon of lime juice
- Salt and black pepper to taste

Sauteed Kale

- 6 cups kale, torn
- 5 teaspoons of olive oil
- dash fine pepper
- 8 teaspoons of pumpkin seeds
- 3 shallots, thinly sliced
- Salt and black pepper to taste

Other Ingredients

- 6 large whole wheat burger buns
- avocado slices

Directions:

1. To make the patties, heat a skillet over medium heat and toast the raw walnuts for about five minutes or until they are golden brown. Spoon the walnuts out of the pan and into a bowl and allow to cool.

2. In the same pan over medium heat, add the olive oil and saute onions until they are translucent. Season with the salt and black pepper. Spoon out of the pan and set aside.
3. Using a blender or food processor, pulse the cooled walnuts with the chili powder, cumin, paprika, light salt, and pepper to taste. Pulse until a fine, grainy texture has been achieved. Set this aside.
4. Mash the dried, cooked black beans with a fork in a large bowl.
5. Add the cooked brown rice, walnut mixture, sauteed onion, bread crumbs, and vegan BBQ sauce. Mix this thoroughly to form a moldable dough. If the mixture is too dry, add more BBQ sauce. If it is too wet, add more breadcrumbs.
6. Divide the dough into six large patties. Press these between your palms to achieve a thickness of ¾ of an inch. Set the prepared patties on a backing sheet or plate.
7. To cook the patties, heat a few drops of olive oil in a large skillet over medium heat. Add as many pantties as can fit in the skillet when hot.
8. Cook for four minutes on each side or until the patties have become well browned.
9. Remove from heat and set aside until time to assemble burgers.
10. While the burgers are cooking make the sauteed kale by heating olive oil in a pan and then adding all the other ingredients to a warm pan. Cover the pot and allow the kale to cook for about one minute. The kale will wilt and become infused with the flavor of the other ingredients. Turn off the heat when down.
11. To make the jalapeno mayo, simply mix all the ingredients in a bowl.
12. Start to assemble the burgers by halving the burger buns and toasting lightly.

13. On one side, spread the jalapeno mayo. Top this with a veggie burger patty then some of the sausted kale. Spread jalapeno mayo on the other bun and close the burger and serve warm.

Crunchy Quinoa Salad with Peanut Sauce

Sweet, spicy, tangy, and good for you, this veggie burger is hearty enough to fuel the rest of your day and flavorful enough to have your taste buds singing. It is packed with anti inflammation ingredients that are easy on your gut.

Nutritional Information

Calcium	93mg
Dietary Fiber	5g
Iron	3mg
Sodium	734mg
Potassium	635mg
Protein	11.2g
Sugars	6.5g
Total Carbohydrates	36.3g
Total Fat	12.2g
Calories per serving	287

Time: 40 minutes

Serving Size: 4

Ingredients:

For Peanut Sauce

- ¼ cup of smooth peanut butter
- 3 tablespoons of soy sauce

- 1 tablespoon of maple syrup
- 1 tablespoon of white vinegar
- 1 teaspoon of olive oil
- 1 teaspoon of grated ginger
- 1 teaspoon of lime juice

For Quinoa Salad

- ¾ cup of washed quinoa
- 1 ½ cups of water
- 2 cups of torn kale
- 1 cup of grated carrot
- ½ cup of chopped cilantro
- ¼ cup of thinly sliced green onion
- ¼ cup of chopped roasted salted peanuts for topping

Directions:

1. Add the washed quinoa to a saucepan and add the oil. Toast the quinoa for a minute and a half over medium heat. The water should completely evaporate.
2. Add water to the lightly toasted quinoa and bring this to a boil.
3. Cook for 15 minutes then turn down the heat to the lowest setting and cover the pot with a lip to make the quinoa fluffy in texture.
4. Remove the quinoa from the heat and let cool. Keep the pot covered for five more minutes. Remove the lid and fluff the quinoa with a fork then set aside to cool further.
5. To make the peanut sauce, microwave peanut butter and soy sauce for 30 seconds that mix for a smooth consistency.
6. Add the remaining ingredients and whisk until smooth. Set aside.
7. In a large bowl, combine the cooled quinoa with the veggies. Toss to combine then add the peanut sauce. Divide the salad and serve.

Mushroom Tofu Sloppy Joes

This recipe makes use of apple cider vinegar, which is a pain reliever for the pain of rheumatoid arthritis. It also reduces the swelling among is anti inflammatory healing properties.

Nutritional Information

Calcium	399mg
Dietary Fiber	7.7g
Iron	5mg
Sodium	501mg
Potassium	775mg
Vitamin D	63mcg
Protein	23.2g
Sugars	6.6g
Total Carbohydrates	26g
Total Fat	24.9g
Calories per serving	391

Time: 40 minutes

Serving Size: 4

Ingredients:

- 4 whole wheat hamburger buns
- 1 cup of grated crimini mushrooms
- 8 ounces firm tofu, drained and crumbled

- 2 tablespoons olive oil
- 1 cup of chopped yellow onion
- 2 tablespoon of sliced garlic
- 2 tablespoons of chili powder
- 1 teaspoon of paprika
- 2 large roasted and pureed tomatoes
- ½ cup finely chopped walnuts
- 2 tablespoons apple cider vinegar
- 2 tablespoons tomato sauce
- 1 tablespoon soy sauce
- Salt to taste

Directions:

1. Heat the olive oil in a large skillet over medium heat and sauté the onion and garlic until the onion becomes translucent.
2. Add mushrooms, tofu, chili powder, and paprika to the skillet. Cook for five minutes, stirring occasionally.
3. Add the roasted pureed tomato purée, walnuts, apple cider vinegar, tomato sauce, and soy sauce.
4. Bring to a boil and then simmer for 15 minutes.
5. Sprinkle with salt and remove from the heat.
6. Slice the buns in half and toast them. Scoop some of the mushroom mixture on the bottom half of the buns and close with the top half.

Green Bean Tofu Salad

Green beans help reduce CRP levels.

Nutritional Information

Calcium	353mg
Dietary Fiber	3.7g
Iron	3mg
Sodium	618mg
Potassium	411mg
Protein	14.8g
Sugars	2g
Total Carbohydrates	7.6g
Total Fat	7.7g
Calories per serving	143

Time: 5 minutes

Serving Size: 4

Ingredients:

- 4 diagonally sliced celery stalks
- 2 cups trimmed and sliced green beans
- ½ braised 8-oz. block firm tofu
- ¼ cup unsalted roasted peanuts
- 2 tablespoon lime juice
- ⅛ teaspoon of salt

Directions:

1. Slice the braised tofu into thin strips.
2. Toss all ingredients together in a medium bowl then serve.

Dinner Recipes

Lemon Chicken Soup

Bay leaf, as used in this recipe, has anti-inflammatory properties that help relieve joint pains and swelling.

Nutritional Information

Calcium	168mg
Dietary Fiber	16.5mg
Iron	9mg
Sodium	231mg
Potassium	1580mg
Protein	83.5g
Sugars	2.5g
Total Carbohydrates	42.5g
Total Fat	34.5g
Calories per serving	823

Time: 45 minutes

Serving Size: 6 (1 ½ cup per serving)

Ingredients:

- 1 pound boneless skinless chicken thighs
- 2 tablespoons of olive oil

- 4 minced cloves of garlic
- 1 diced yellow pepper
- 1 cup of diced carrots
- 2 diced celery stalks
- half a teaspoon of dried thyme
- 8 cups of unsalted chicken stock
- 2 cups of cooked cannellini beans
- 1 cups of spinach
- 2 tablespoons of lemon juice
- 2 tablespoons of chopped parsley
- 2 tbsp of chopped dill
- 2 bay leaves
- Salt and pepper to taste

Directions:

1. Cut the chicken into one-inch chunks and season with salt and pepper.
2. In a large Dutch oven, heat one tablespoon of olive oil the medium heat. Sear the chicken on both sides until golden brown then set aside.
3. Add the remaining olive oil to the Dutch oven then saute the garlic, onion, celery, and carrots. Stir occasionally and cook the vegetables until tender. Stir in the thyme for about a minute.
4. And the bay leaves and chicken stock and bring the mixture to a boil.
5. Reduce the heat and stir in cannellini beans and chicken. Stir occasionally and cook this for 15 minutes or until the gravy has thickened slightly.
6. Add the spinach and cook for about two minutes.
7. Stir in remaining ingredients.
8. Remove from heat and serve immediately.

Curried Veggies Over Brown Rice

Nutritional Information

Calcium	140mg
Dietary Fiber	12.4g
Iron	7mg
Sodium	332mg
Potassium	1192mg
Protein	18.8g
Sugars	8.6g
Total Carbohydrates	166g
Total Fat	30.8g
Calories per serving	996

Time: 15 minutes

Serving Size: 4

Ingredients:

- 4 cups of cooked brown rice
- 1 tablespoon of olive oil
- 1 cup of chopped yellow onion
- 1 tablespoon of grated ginger
- 1 tablespoon of minced garlic
- 1 red bell pepper, sliced into thin 2-inch long strips
- 1 green bell pepper, sliced into thin long strips
- 3 julienned carrot

- 2 tablespoons of curry powder
- 1 ½ cup of coconut milk
- ½ cup water
- 1 ½ cups of spinach
- 1 tablespoon of soy sauce
- 2 teaspoons of lime juice
- Chopped basil for topping
- Salt to taste

Directions:

1. To make the curry, heat the olive oil in a large skillet over medium heat and sauté the onions until translucent. Add the garlic and ginger and cook for 30 seconds while stirring.
2. Add carrots and bell peppers and cook until the peppers are tender. Sti occasionally.
3. Add the curry powder and stir. cook for two minutes.
4. Add the coconut milk, water and spinach and stir to combine. Bring to a boil over medium heat then simmer for seven minutes. Stir occasionally.
5. Remove the curry from heat and add the lime juice and salt.
6. Divide the brown rice between four bowls and top with curried vegetables. Garnish with basil and serve warm.

Garlic-Infused Seared Scallops

Scallops are rich in omega-3 fatty acids, making it a great anti inflammatory food. It is also a great source of protein.

Nutritional Information

Calcium	12mg
Dietary Fiber	0.1g
Sodium	61mg
Potassium	134mg
Protein	6.4g
Sugars	0.1g
Total Carbohydrates	1.2g
Total Fat	3.8g
Calories per serving	64

Time: 15 minutes

Serving Size: 4

Ingredients:

- 1 pound large scallops
- 1 tablespoon olive oil
- 2 tbsp. freshly chopped parsley
- Salt and black pepper to taste
- Lemon wedges

Directions:

1. Over medium heat, heat the olive oil in a large skillet. Saute the garlic.
2. Blot the scallops dry with paper towels to prevent oil splatter that can lead to injury. Season the scallops with salt and pepper.
3. Add the scallops to the heated oil mixture.
4. Cook the scallops until the bottom gets a golden crust. This will take about two minutes. Flip and cook until the same happens to the other side.
5. Serve scallops over veggies, cooked brown rice or cooked quinoa. Squeeze the lemon wedges over.

Maple Garlic Salmon

High in omega-3 fatty acids, salmon decreases CRP levels.

Nutritional Information

Calcium	84mg
Dietary Fiber	0.2g
Iron	2mg
Sodium	960mg
Potassium	733mg
Protein	34.2g
Sugars	16.9g
Total Carbohydrates	19.7g
Total Fat	21.1g
Calories per serving	394

Time: 25 minutes

Serving Size: 4

Ingredients:

- 4 6-oz. salmon fillets
- ⅓ cups of maple syrup
- ¼ cups of low-sodium soy sauce
- 2 tablespoon lemon juice
- 3 tablespoon olive oil
- 1 tablespoon minced garlic
- Lemon slices

- Salt and black pepper to taste
- Freshly chopped parsley for topping

Directions:

1. In a medium bowl, whisk together maple, soy sauce, and lemon juice.
2. In a large skillet over medium heat, heat two tablespoons oil. Add the salmon, which has been blotted with paper towels to remove the excess moisture, skin-side up. season with salt and pepper.
3. Cook the salmon for five minutes or until deeply golden.
4. Flip over and add remaining tablespoon of oil. Add garlic to skillet and cook for a minute.
5. Add the maple mixture and sliced lemons and cook until the sauce becomes reduced by about one-third. Baste the salmon with the sauce.
6. Top with parsley and serve.

Pan Fried Tuna

Tuna is another fish that is high in omega-3 fatty acids, thus its great anti inflammatory benefits.

Nutritional Information

Calcium	90mg
Dietary Fiber	8.4g
Iron	7mg
Sodium	207mg
Potassium	1550mg
Protein	125.3g
Sugars	0.5g
Total Carbohydrates	9.7g
Total Fat	38.7g
Calories per serving	894

Time: 25 minutes

Serving Size: 4

Ingredients:

- 4 6-oz. tuna fillets
- 1 cup of flax meal (grounded flax seeds)
- 1 teaspoon of garlic powder
- 1 teaspoon of onion powder
- 1 teaspoon of chili powder
- ½ teaspoon of ground cumin

- 1 tablespoon of canola oil
- Salt and black pepper to taste
- Lemon wedges, for serving
- Freshly chopped parsley for topping

Directions:

1. Combine the flax meal, garlic powder, onion powder, chili powder, and ground cumin in a large bowl.
2. Season the tuna fillets with salt and pepper. Dip them in the flax meal mixture then shake off any excess before placing each on a baking tray.
3. Heat the canola oil in a large nonstick skillet over medium heat. Add as many tuna fillets as the skillet can hold without crowding. Cook on each side for about three minutes or until golden brown. Repeat with any remaining tuna fillets.
4. Serve with lemon wedges and chopped parsley.

Kale Stuffed Sardines with Roasted Carrot Sticks

This recipe is great because of the omega-3 fatty acids in the sardines and the kale.

Nutritional Information

Calcium	337mg
Dietary Fiber	1.6g
Iron	3mg
Sodium	402mg
Potassium	616mg
Protein	19.9g
Sugars	1.6g
Total Carbohydrates	11g
Total Fat	18.2g
Calories per serving	283

Time: 25 minutes

Serving Size: 4

Ingredients:

- 2 cups shredded kale
- 1 cup boiling water
- 2 tablespoons of raisins
- 2 tablespoons of pine nuts

- 1 crushed garlic clove
- ½ teaspoon of finely grated lemon zest
- 12 cleaned sardines
- 2 tablespoons of olive oil
- 1 tablespoon freshly chopped parsley
- 2 tablespoon of panko bread crumbs
- Roasted carrot sticks, for serving (see recipe in Snacks Section)

Directions:

1. Preheat your oven to 400 degrees F.
2. Prepare a baking sheet with parchment paper.
3. Put kale in a heatproof bowl and cover with boiling water. Allow this to stand for one minute before draining the water. Refresh the kale under cold running water. Squeeze to remove excess liquid.
4. Place kale in a food processor with raisins, pine nuts, garlic, and lemon zest, and pulse to a rough texture.
5. Stuff the cavity of the sardines with the kale mixture, then place on the baking tray.
6. Sprinkle the sardines with bread crumbs then drizzle with olive oil. Bake for 15 minutes or until golden brown.
7. Serve the baked sardines over the roasted carrot sticks and sprinkle with chopped parsley.

Maple Roasted Salmon

Nutritional Information

Calcium	
Calcium	63mg
Iron	1mg
Sodium	103mg
Potassium	663g
Protein	33g
Sugars	2g
Total Carbohydrates	2.5g
Total Fat	11.4g
Calories per serving	243

Time: 25 minutes

Serving Size: 4

Ingredients:

- 4 6-oz salmon fillets
- 2 tablespoons finely chopped fresh cilantro
- 1 tablespoon vegan mayonnaise
- 2 teaspoons maple syrup
- Salt and black pepper to taste

Directions:

1. Preheat your oven to 400 degrees F.

2. Line a baking sheet with aluminium foil. Place the salmon fillets on top.
3. In a small bowl, combine the cilantro, mayonnaise, and maple syrup. Spread this mixture on top of the salmon fillets and sprinkle with salt and pepper.
4. Bake for 11 minutes.

Garnish with some chopped cilantro and serve.

CPSIA information can be obtained
at www.ICGtesting.com
Printed in the USA
BVHW041740310121
599088BV00014B/24

9 781801 380669